Medical Face Mask

Photos inside: A Quick and Practical Guide on How to Build Your Mask at Home and in an Emergency Situation To Protect You From Viruses and Bacteria

Ariel Walker

© Copyright 2020 by Ariel Walker. All right reserved.

The work contained herein has been produced with the intent to provide relevant knowledge and information on the topic described in the title for entertainment purposes only. While the author has gone to every extent to furnish up to date and true information, no claims can be made as to its accuracy or validity as the author has made no claims to be an expert on this topic. Notwithstanding, the reader is asked to do their own research and consult any subject matter experts they deem necessary to ensure the quality and accuracy of the material presented herein.

This statement is legally binding as deemed by the Committee of Publishers Association and the American Bar Association for the territory of the United States. Other jurisdictions may apply their own legal statutes. Any reproduction, transmission or copying of this material contained in this work without the express written consent of the copyright holder shall be deemed as a copyright violation as per the current legislation in force on the date of publishing and subsequent time thereafter. All additional works derived from this material may be claimed by the holder of this copyright.

The data, depictions, events, descriptions and all other information forthwith are considered to be true, fair and accurate unless the work is expressly described as a work of fiction. Regardless of the nature of this work, the Publisher is exempt from any responsibility of actions taken by the reader in conjunction with this work. The Publisher acknowledges that the reader acts of their own accord and releases the author and Publisher of any responsibility for the observance of tips, advice, counsel, strategies and techniques that may be offered in this volume.

Table of Contents

Introduction
Chapter 1: What Is a Face Mask

   Mask Classification
   Certifications

Chapter 2: When Masks Should Be Used

   What Diseases Can Face Masks Prevent the Spread of?

Chapter 3: Mask Etiquette

   When to Wear Masks
   What the CDC Says About Cloth Masks
   Wearing a Cloth Mask
   Putting on a Surgical Mask
   Things You Shouldn't Do When Wearing a Mask
   Removing and Throwing Away the Mask
   The Best Way to Limit Infections

Chapter 4: Making Your Own Mask

   Sewn Cloth Face Mask
   No Sew Mask
   Quick T-Shirt Mask

Chapter 5: Making an Emergency Mask

   Emergency Cleaning Cloth Face Mask
   Emergency Coffee Filter Mask

Chapter 6: Where to Purchase Face Masks
Chapter 7: Other Ways to Protect Yourself

   You Have to Know How Infections Get Transmitted
   Good Hygiene
   Practice Food Safety
   Vaccinations Are Essential
   Travel Precautions
   Sexually Transmitted Infections
   Animal Control
   Coronavirus or COVID-19
   Everybody Needs to

Conclusion

Introduction

First off, I would like to thank you for choosing this book, and I hope that you find the information within informative. Faces masks use to not be something that was talked about regularly. They were something that medical professionals wore. But then things change and we experience something like SAR or COVID-19 and face masks become our new normal.

The other issue when things like this happen is sometimes things become hard to find. When you need a face mask to protect yourself and others, but can't find one, what are you supposed to do? Make one yourself, of course. That's what we are going to discuss in this book.

First, though, we will discuss what a face mask is, as well as the different types of face masks. Some are for professional use, and others are made for the general public, and there is a big difference between the two.

Then we'll discuss when masks should be used. Sometimes it is easy to overreact to things, which could cause us to use a face mask when we don't necessarily need one, or we don't use one when we should. So we will clear up this confusion with clear cut reasons why a face mask should be worn.

We will then move into mask etiquette. Even though they seem like simple things to wear, there is a proper way to wear, remove, and dispose of face masks.

After that, you will find the chapter that likely drew you to this book. We will go over three different ways to make your own face mask. These will be regular, cloth face masks that the general public can use if need be. Then we'll go over two ways to make an emergency face mask. These can help you if you are out in public and suddenly realize you need one and don't have one available to you.

Next, we'll go over various places where you may be able to purchase face masks. This isn't information that the general public likely has because we aren't faced with the need to have and wear face masks on a regular basis.

Lastly, we'll discuss other ways to protect yourself from disease and illness. Faces masks should not be your be all end all choice of safety when it comes to disease prevention. There are other things you can do that can increase your safety during cold and flu season or a pandemic.

Medical Disclaimer

Before we begin, it's important to understand that I am not a health care provider, so the information in this book should not be considered medical advice. It is just helpful information that you can refer to if need be, and should not be used as a substitute for seeing an actual doctor.

With that in mind, let's begin.

Chapter 1: What Is a Face Mask

A face mask is, normally, a disposable, loose-fitting device that forms a physical barrier between the nose and mouth of the wearer and any possible contaminants in their environment. If they are worn correctly, they will help to block large-particle droplets, splatter, sprays, or splashes that could contain bacteria and viruses, keeping it from coming in contact from the wearer's nose and mouth.

There are various types of face masks. The first type is the surgical mask. These are the disposable masks worn by surgeons and other hospital personnel to prevent cross contamination during surgeries and other health care procedures. They keep microorganisms from the wearer's nose and mouth from falling into wounds or sores. The surgical mask also helps remind the wearer not to touch their nose and mouth, which could end up transferring bacteria and viruses.

By design, surgical masks do not block or filter very small particles in the air that could be transmitted through sneezes, coughs, or some medical procedures. Surgical masks are not able to provide complete protection from germs because they fit loosely between the skin and the mask.

We also have cloth face masks, which are a semi-recent creation, and are reusable. With the face mask shortage, the world has faced with the COVID-19 pandemic, people have turned to creating their own face masks as a form of protection. They are created from cloth, whereas surgical masks are made from nonwoven fabric formed through a melt blowing process. Cloth face masks are not regulated, and they also do not form a seal around the face.

They are mainly used on patients who are already sick as a form of "source control" in order to reduce the transmission of disease. They can also be worn by healthcare workers when surgical masks are unavailable. With that said, let's move into the different classifications for face masks.

Mask Classification

There are three main levels of face mask classifications.

1. Procedure masks/Level 1

The first is the procedure mask. These are easily identified by their two ear loops that secure the mask to your face. These are mainly only used on the hospital floor, in isolation units, and in the labor and delivery units. They may also be used in the emergency room and intensive care. However, they are not approved from use in the operating room. They are typically single use and have one thin layer. They are only effective at stopping the spread of larger dust particles

2. Surgical masks/Level 2

These are the masks used by the OR staff and typically have four straps, one from each corner, that are tied around the head to secure them. They do not have the ear loops because a tighter seal can be formed from the ties than loops can. They are mean to protect against high-risk fluid exposure. They are created for sterile environments, whereas procedure masks are not. They have higher requirements for the particles they can capture, but these requirements vary by country.

3. Respirators/Level 3

The most common respirator is the N95. These are used to filter surgical smoke that is formed from devices like electrosurgical units or ultrasonic scalpels that are using during invasive procedures. N95 respirators are also recommended for health care personnel when they are at a higher risk of exposure to aerosol-transmittable diseases, like rubella, tuberculosis, and varicella.

Certifications

In the US, face masks are tested and rated by the American Society of Testing and Materials, ASTM. In Europe, they are tested by European Standards and are marked with a CE.

According to the ASTM, there are five main categories that a face mask can be rated for. First is the bacterial filtration efficiency. This is how well the mask can filter out bacteria. For surgical masks, they need to have a 95% filtration rate.

The second category is particulate filtration efficiency. This is how well the mask filters small particles, such as viruses. Then they look at the fluid resistance. This is basically how well the inner layer protects from spray or splashes.

The fourth category is its pressure differential. This is basically how breathable the mask is. Lastly, they look at flammability. Surgery rooms have a high potential for fire due to oxygen and other gases. Surgical masks should be able to withstand exposure to flame for three seconds.

Every level of mask undergoes these tests. Level 1 masks are the only mask that does not require a particulate filtration efficiency.

In the US, surgical masks are labeled as ASTM F2100. In Europe, they are labeled EN 14683. While we won't get into the details of each, these surgical masks are also broken down into three different levels of protection.

When it comes to respirator masks, in the US, they are regulated by NIOSH. There are seven different types of respirators, most of which are not used for disease control, but are used by professionals who work in bad air quality, such as firefighters and auto mechanics. The different types of respirator masks are:

- N95 – This is the only respirator mask that has been developed and approved by the FDA for use as a surgical or healthcare mask
- N99
- N100

- R95
- P95
- P99
- P100

In Europe, their N95 counterpart is the EN 149:2001.

As you can see, there are a lot of different types of face masks, all of which have their own purpose and use. As far as face mask use among the general public, it is recommended that they only use the procedure or cloth face masks.

Chapter 2: When Masks Should Be Used

As humans, we naturally like to be prepared for anything. This means using face masks or other protective measures to protect ourselves from diseases. The problem is, we can sometimes use masks or the likes when we don't really need to. The Us Surgeon General, CDC, and other health care advisors recommend that people refrain from using face masks unless they are exhibiting symptoms. The main reason they suggest this is to make sure that hospitals and other health care providers don't experience a shortage in their supplies. They also believe that these face masks to little good at preventing a person from developing certain illnesses. However, the issue here is that there are very few studies performed on how effective face masks are against respiratory infections.

Generally speaking, if you know that you are going to be somewhere where you could be exposed to an illness, or you're worried you could be asymptomatic, you should wear only a cloth face mask. The use of surgical masks should be limited to healthcare workers, people who know they are infected, or people are taking care of a person who is infected.

N95 respirator masks should never be used by the general public. They are needed in health care facilities where they are supposed to be used.

Now, these recommendations and regulations can defer in other countries. People in areas like Japan, Thailand, and Chine will often reuse disposable surgical masks. This is not good practice and increases a person's risk of infection. They are disposable masks for a reason.

Also, in many Asian countries, wearing a face mask is something that is done as a hygienic practice. That means they will likely be wearing a face mask, whether there is a known health risk or not because of air quality. Whereas, in North America and Europe, face masks are only used by those who feel unwell. This has caused a bit of stigma for people in North American and European countries. If somebody decided to wear a face mask because they knew they were sick, they would likely be judged more harshly by others than a person in an Asian country would. This is what makes it so hard to decide whether or not you should wear a face mask.

Some basic guidelines for when it is appropriate to wear a face mask are:

- When you are going to be within six feet of a person who is ill.

- When you will be in a setting where you can't easily stay six feet away from people who may be ill.

- When you, yourself, are ill and will around others who are healthy.

In general, if you are healthy and are not exhibiting any signs of disease and you are able to stay six feet or farther away from others, you do not necessarily need to wear a face mask. That said, if you want to be on the safe side, wearing a homemade cloth face mask is your best bet. This will protect you and others to a certain extent without taking away surgical masks from those who absolutely need them.

What Diseases Can Face Masks Prevent the Spread of?

For the most part, in countries like the US, people don't think about wearing face masks unless there is a perceived threat. As such, this makes us leery of their efficacy because we don't see them being used in public often. But, masks can be helpful in preventing the spread of any respiratory disease.

A 2013 study found that wearing a face mask during the time when the seasonal flu is most prevalent can help limit the spread of the disease. The researchers found that face masks led to a more than threefold reduction in how many virus particles were in the air.

Face masks can also reduce the spread of other flu viruses, such as H1N1 and H5N1. They can also help reduce a person's risk of catching the common cold, and they are also used to prevent the spread of SARS and MERS in Asian countries.

But faces masks are just effective when it comes to reducing the spread of viruses. They can also help to reduce the spread of bacterial infections as well. The spread of pneumonia can be reduced through the use of a face mask as well. It has also been proven that face masks can slow the spread of diseases like tuberculosis, ebola, varicella, streptococcus, and measles.

That said, there are just as many, if not more, diseases that can't be prevented through a face mask. Bacterial and fungal diseases tend to be the trickiest illnesses to prevent, but they are also easier to combat because there are more drugs that can be used to fight them off. Viruses can't be helped with medications like antibiotics, and have to be left to run its course, which is why viruses tend to be more deadly.

All diseases, no matter what they are caused by, can be transmitted to other people. Some are more easily transmitted than others. Those that are spread through aerosol particles, such as mucus and saliva, are the types of diseases that can be contained through the use of a face mask to a certain extent.

If the disease does not create respiratory symptoms, then they cannot as easily be contained using face masks. For example, STIs are only able to be transmitted through sex, or exposure to their blood. Hepatitis is another disease that can only be transmitted through contact with blood or fecal matter, and can't be easily spread through airborne mucus or saliva.

If you do have a fever or respiratory symptoms, then wearing a cloth face mask when out in public is a good idea. If you aren't sure, then the best thing to do is to talk to your doctor.

Chapter 3: Mask Etiquette

Wearing face masks can help people feel reassured and protected. Could surgical masks keep you from transmitting or being exposed to specific diseases?

If a face mask can protect you from an infectious disease like COVID-19, is there a right way to put them on, remove them, and then throw them away? Let's find out.

If a surgical mask can help block microorganisms from being transmitted from person to person through splashes, splatters, sprays, and droplets, it could reduce hand-to-face contact.

A surgical mask's layers help in this manner:

- The outside will repel bodily fluids, blood, and water.
- The center can filter out specific pathogens.
- The inside absorbs the sweat and moisture from the air that is exhaled.

The main drawback of these masks is that the edges won't form a tight-fitting seal around the mouth or nose. This means that they aren't able to filter out small particles like those that are transmitted through sneezing and coughing.

When to Wear Masks

The WHO or World Health Organization says you need to wear a mask if you:

- Feel fine, but you care for somebody that has a respiratory illness. If this is the case, you need to wear a mask anytime you are near the person who is sick. "Near" refers to being within six feet.
- Have any respiratory symptoms, a cough, or a fever.

Even though surgical masks can trap bigger droplets, it won't protect you from catching this new coronavirus, which is also called SARS-CoV-2. This is because a surgical mask:

- Won't fit tightly against the face. This allows small particles to leak through the mask's sides.
- Can't filter out the tiny airborne particles

There have been studies that show surgical masks can keep you from being exposed to diseases in public or community settings.

At the present time, the CDC or Centers for Disease Control and Prevention, isn't recommending that the public wear masks to protect them from illnesses such as the new COVID-19. First responders and healthcare providers are in need of these supplies, and there is a shortage at this time.

The CDC is recommending that the public wear a cloth face covering to keep the disease from spreading. You can find instructions in a later chapter on how to make your own.

What the CDC Says About Cloth Masks

The CDC does recommend that you wear a cloth face mask in public where you aren't able to social distance yourself from others like pharmacies or grocery stores, especially in tight areas like registers.

The CDC also recommends that using simple cloth masks can slow the spread of viruses that can help people who might already have the virus but just don't know it from spreading it to other people. Cloth masks that are made from items found in the home can be used voluntarily by the public.

Cloth face masks should never be put on children under the age of two, anybody who has breathing problems, or anyone who is incapacitated or unconscious and can't remove it without help.

The cloth face masks that are recommended aren't the N95s or surgical masks. These are critical supplies that need to be reserved for first responders and healthcare workers.

Wearing a Cloth Mask

A cloth mask needs to:

- Include more than one layer of fabric
- Fit comfortably and snugly against the face
- Have the ability to be machine washed and dried without changing its shape or damaging the mask
- Be tied behind the neck or have ear loops
- Allow you to breathe without any obstructions

The instructions below on how to put a surgical mask on needs to be done for a cloth mask, too.

Putting on a Surgical Mask

If you have to wear a mask, do the following steps so you can wear it properly:

1. Before you put the mask on, you need to thoroughly wash your hands for 20 seconds. Make sure you use water and soap. You could also use hand sanitizer if you don't have access to water and soap.

2. Look at the mask and see if you can notice any defects like broken loops or tears.

3. Place the side that is colored to the outside.

4. If the mask has one, place the metal strip located at the top of the mask against the bridge of your nose.

5. Depending on what the mask has:

    a. Dual elastic bands: you need to pull the band on the top over the head and put it on the crown of the head. Now pull the band on the bottom over the head and put it at the back of the neck.

    b. Ties: Place the top strings in your hands and tie them in a bow close to the crown. Now tie the strings on the bottom in a bow at the back of the neck.

    c. Ear loops: by holding the mask by both loops and put a loop around each ear.

6. Now you need to bend that metal strip to fit your nose snuggly. You can do this by pressing down and pinching it with your thumb and forefinger.

7. Place the bottom part of the mask up and over your chin and mouth.

8. Make sure the mask is fitting snuggly.

9. Never touch your mask once you have it on.

10. Once the mask gets damp or soiled, put a new one on as soon as you possibly can.

Things You Shouldn't Do When Wearing a Mask

When you have the mask placed properly, there are some precautions you have to remember to make sure you don't transfer any pathogens to your hands or face.

NEVER:

- Reuse a mask that is disposable
- Cross the ties
- Hang it around the neck
- Allow the mask to hang from one ear
- Touch it after you have it secured to your face because it could have pathogens on it.

If you absolutely need to touch your mask once it is on, wash or sanitize the hands first. Make sure you wash or sanitize your hands after you touch it, too.

Removing and Throwing Away the Mask

It is important that you remove your mask correctly to make sure you aren't transferring any germs to your face or hands. You need to make sure you throw away the mask properly.

How to take the mask off:

1. Wash or sanitize your hands before you remove the mask.
2. DON'T touch the mask since it might be contaminated. Make sure you only touch it by the bands, ties, or loops.
3. Remove the mask carefully after you have:
    a. Taken off each ear loop or
    b. Untie the bow on the bottom first and then until the one on top or
    c. Take off the band on the bottom first by pulling it up and over the head, do this with the band on top, too.
4. Hold the mask by the bands, ties, or loops throw the mask away by putting it into a trash bin that is covered.
5. Once you have taken the mask off, wash or sanitize your hands.

The Best Way to Limit Infections

The best way to minimize transmitting a respiratory illness to others is to stay away from them. This also applies if you want to avoid getting a virus.

The WHO recommends the following to reduce your chances of coming into contact or transmitting any virus:

- Stay home and get plenty of rest
- Stay away from the public until you have completely recovered
- Stay at least six feet from other people
- DON'T touch your eyes, mouth, and face
- If you can't get to water and soap, use hand sanitizer that is at least 60% alcohol
- Wash your hands frequently using water and soap for no less than 20 seconds

Bottom Line

Masks could protect you from large particles that get airborne, but the N95 does give you more protection from the small airborne particles.

Placing the masks on your face and removing them the right way can protect you and the people around you from getting or transmitting pathogens.

Even though face masks could help reduce spreading certain diseases, evidence says that face masks might not protect you from being exposed to specific pathogens.

FAQs

1. Should a cloth mask be washed or cleaned on a regular basis, and how often?

Absolutely. They need to be washed after each use.

2. How can you safely clean or sanitize a cloth mask?

Washing the cloth masks in a washing machine will sanitize and clean the cloth mask.

3. How can you safely take off a cloth face mask?

Wash or sanitize your hands before you take off the mask. Make sure you don't touch your mouth, nose, or eyes when you take off the mask. Wash or sanitize your hands right after you take off the mask.

Chapter 4: Making Your Own Mask

We all know that there is a shortage of N95 respirators and surgical masks right now, but what can you do when you want to go out but want to protect yourself from germs?

Well, the first thing to know is that masks aren't mandatory yet they are just recommended.

Homemade masks aren't ever a substitute for staying at home or staying away from others.

If you would like to make a mask, here are a few simple ways you can make a mask. Don't worry about it if you don't know how to sew as I have included instructions for a couple that don't require any sewing.

Just remember to clean your mask after each wear.

Sewn Cloth Face Mask

The time it takes to make this mask will vary according to your sewing skill. This is an intermediate skill level sewing craft.

What you will need:

- Sewing machine
- Scissors
- Bobby pin or needle and thread
- 6 inch elastic pieces, 2
- 10 inch X 6 inch pieces of cotton fabric, 2

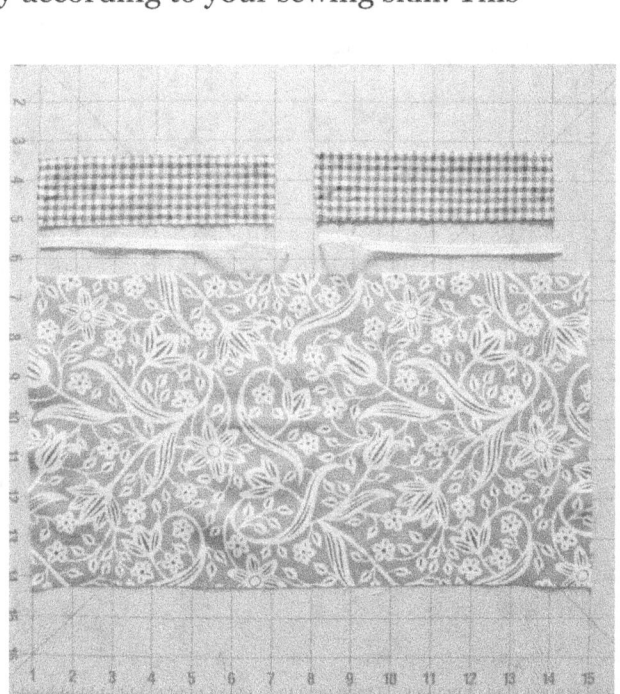

What you will do:

Cut the two 10 X 6 inch rectangles from the cotton fabric. Try to use cotton that is tightly woven like sheets or quilting fabric. An old pair of jeans would work well, too.

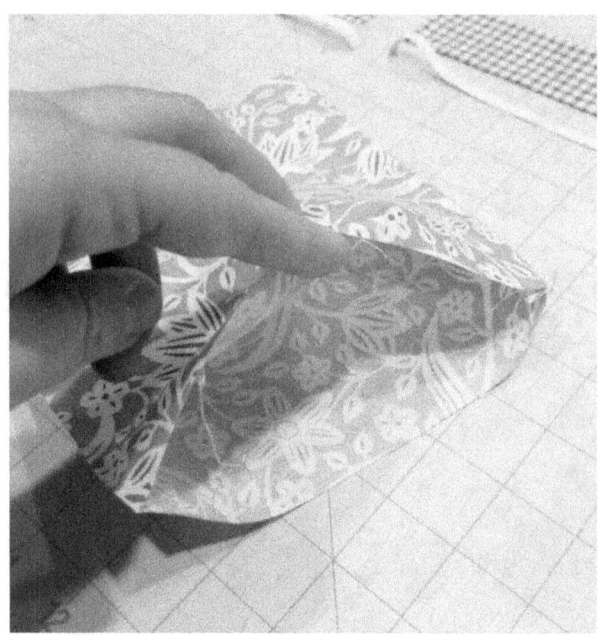

Take the long sides and fold over a quarter inch and stitch this. Do this for the other side, too. Now fold the doubled fabric over one half inch on the short sides and sew this down on each side.

Take a six inch length of elastic through the larger him on the short ends of the mask. These are going to be the loops that go around the ears. You can use the bobby pin to help you get the elastic through. Tie the ends together.

If you don't have any elastic, you can use elastic head bands or hair ties. You will just need to cut them so you can fit them through the openings. If you just have strings, you can use longer ties and tie the mask behind the head.

Slowly pull the elastic around, so the knots are inside the hem. Gather the mask on the elastic sides and adjust it to fit your face. Stitch the elastic in place at the corners of the mask so it won't slip.

Slip the ear loops over your ears, and you have just sewn your very own face mask.

No-Sew Mask

This is an easy mask to make if you don't have sewing materials or just don't have the time to sew. You just need a piece of material that is 20 inches by 20 inches. If you are a stickler for getting things exactly perfect, you might want to have a ruler on hand. Some people find it easier to iron the sides down as you fold them to make them stay in place better.

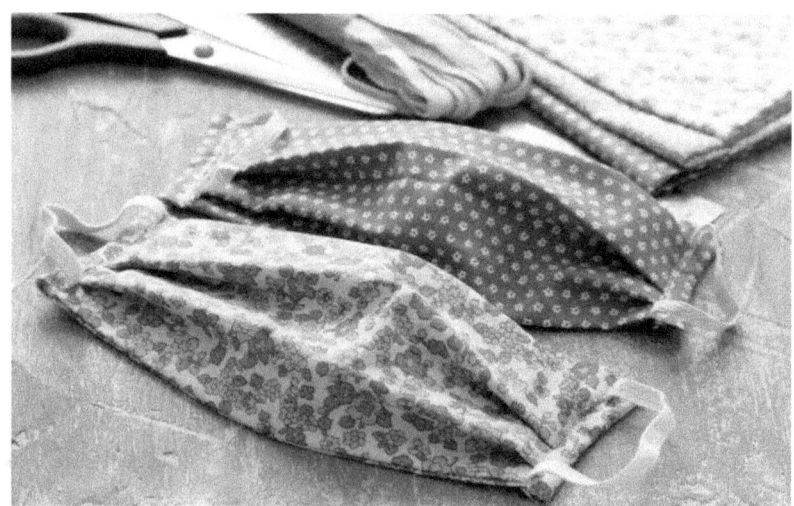

The time it will take you to make this mask will vary, but it shouldn't take longer than ten minutes. This is an easy project that would make a fun project for children to do when they get bored.

What you will need:

- Hair ties or rubber bands
- Coffee filter
- 20 X 20 inch square cloth, cotton, T-shirt, or bandana
- Scissors

What you will do:

Take a coffee filter and fold it in half. Cut the bottom part off. You will need the top parts for the mask.

Lay your 20 X 20 piece of material down flat. Fold it in half to make a rectangle.

Place the top half of the coffee filter into the center of this rectangle. Now, fold the top third of the cloth down over the coffee filter and the bottom third up over the coffee filter.

Put the hair ties or rubber bands around the folded cloth where they are about six inches from each other.

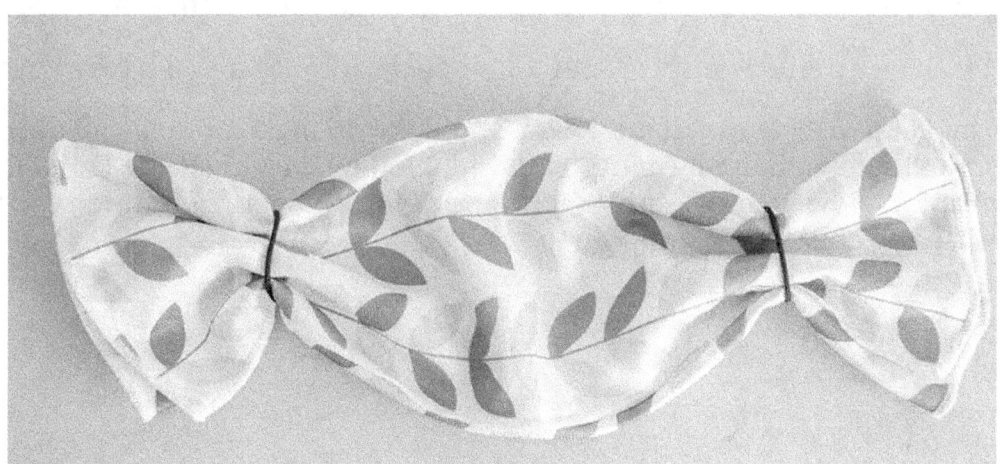

Now, you are going to fold the sides of the cloth in toward the center and tuck the ends into each other.

Slip the rubber bands around your ears, and you have made a new sew face mask.

Quick T-Shirt Mask

This is a great craft to do that will use up some of those old T-shirts that you have stuffed into a drawer. No sewing required; all you are going to need is a pair of scissors and a ruler. This shouldn't take you any longer than about ten minutes to do. You can even do this with your child's old T-shirts, too. That way they have a mask that won't be too large for their face. Remember that it isn't recommended for a child under the age of two to wear a face mask.

You are going to need:

- Scissors

- T-shirt
- Ruler
- Sharpie or other marker

You are going to do:

Take the ruler and measure eight inches up from the bottom of the T-shirt. Mark this with the marker.

Cut across the line you just made.

Now, take the ruler and measure a half inch from the bottom and top of the piece you just cut. Make a small mark. Now use the ruler to measure six inches in from one side. You need to mark a rectangular shape that is half an inch from the top and bottom and six inches in from the side. Cut this out.

Now, you need to cut the thin strips on one side so that they look like ties.

Tie these around your neck and top of the head so that you have a mask.

You get to decide which mask you would like to make or make all of them and share them with family and friends. Just follow the guidelines listed in the chapter above to make sure you keep your mask clean and sanitary. Remember to wash the mask every time you use it.

Chapter 5: Making an Emergency Mask

There may be times when you are out and about, and you realize that you need a face mask. For whatever reason, you could find yourself walking down the street or through a grocery and suddenly realize that you need a face mask. You check your purse, your car, your pocket, or whatever you have with you, but you don't have anything on you, or at least that's what you think.

There are ways to make quick and easy emergency face masks. The two emergency masks we are going to go over do not require sewing, which is important for an emergency face mask, and will use items that you will likely be able to easily get when you are out.

Emergency Cleaning Cloth Face Mask

This is a quick and easy face mask that you can make using things that you will likely be able to easily find in a store or in your car.

You are going to need:

- Stapler
- 2 hair elastics
- A thick square cleaning cloth/paper towel

You are going to do:

The paper towel or cleaning cloth that you will need are like some of the paper towels that you can find in some public restrooms. You shouldn't use the brown paper towels or the thinner ones; they won't last. Shop towels are similar to the thickness you need for this.

Once you have located the paper towel you need, lay it out flat on a clean and sanitized surface. You will create an accordion fold with the paper towel so that it resembles a face mask. You will make about three folds.

Then you will take your stapler and staple both ends of the towel so that the accordion folds do not come undone.

Next, you will take one of your hair elastics and slip it over one end of the mask. Fold the end over the elastic and use your stapler to staple it closed so that the hair elastic is a container in the towel. Do the same thing with the other hair elastic on the other end of the mask.

Now all you have to do is slip the hair elastics over your ears, and you have a mask.

Emergency Coffee Filter Mask

This one will only take one ingredient and is something that most mothers will have with them. If not, they can easily be found in stores.

You are going to need:

- 3 baby wipes

It's a good idea to use the thicker baby wipes that aren't easily ripped to make sure that this one holds up.

All you need to do is to lay the three baby wipes, one on top of each other. At one end, fold the end over about a quarter of an inch. Then, using scissors, cut the middle part of the edge you have created off. Basically, once you unfold this edge, you should have a hole that will slip over your ear.

Do the same thing on the other end of the baby wipes. Next, all you need to do is to slip the two holes over your ears to wear this as a mask. This mask will smell like baby wipes, so if you are sensitive to smells, this may not be the best option. Also, you will want to let the wipes dry out a bit.

Chapter 6: Where to Purchase Face Masks

If you aren't much of a sewer, or you have time to wait on getting your masks, you can also buy face masks. Creating your own face mask isn't for everybody, and that's perfectly okay. If you still want to help stop the spread of communicable diseases, however, there are places where you can purchase premade, nonmedical face masks.

Once again, these are nonmedical face masks. All medical face masks should be used by medical personnel or those who are already ill. So, let's look at where you can purchase your own cloth face coverings.

When you start shopping around for your face mask, make sure that look for one's that are being created from cotton and come with a filter pouch. Ones that are pleated will offer you more layers. You should make sure that the mask is wide enough to cover your chin and nose, and that is should be snug enough where there are no gaps. Making sure it has a tight fit will help to keep out large particles that move throughout the air from things like sneezes.

When you receive your purchased face mask, you should make sure that you wash it before you use it. It is best if you purchase multiple masks so that you will always have a clean one on hand when you need it because your mask should be washed once you get home.

It's also important to remember that just because you are wearing a nonmedical face mask does not mean you shouldn't follow other hygienic practices, such as social and physical distancing and hand washing. Also, it is always good to remember that just because you are wearing a face mask, does not mean that you won't be able to catch an illness or disease, but it will reduce your chance.

Without further ado, here are a few different places where you can find cloth face masks.

- Custom Ink

Custom Ink is a printing company that specializes in customized gear for groups and businesses. Since the COVID-19 pandemic, they have now started to use their resources to manufacture protective cloth face masks. They offer a family 12 pack for only $30. They clearly state that the masks are for personal use only and should not be worn by people in a clinical or surgical setting where the risk for infection is high.

- Facebook Marketplace

If you know that you can safely purchase a homemade face mask from a person that is local, then Facebook Marketplace would be a good place to find them. If, when you are purchasing your face masks, there is a need for social distancing, make sure that you remain at least six feet aware from them. That means you should make sure that you make arrangements to take the items of their porch or see if they are willing to ship them to you.

- Etsy

Etsy is a popular choice for purchasing homemade items. It is also a great place to buy multiple face masks in several different patterns. They will also sell out fairly quickly, so you may have to check back often. Some Etsy stores will also offer free shipping when you purchase $35 or more. There are even some sellers that carry adult and children sizes, so make sure that you check the sizes. You'd hate to wind up with a kids size mask.

The great thing with Etsy is that they require their sellers to be transparent about their process and standards for creating a face mask. For example, none of them can be labeled as a medical device since they are not medical grade. They are also unable to advertise their masks as being able to prevent, mitigate, treat, cure, or diagnose any health condition or disease.

- Arm The Animals

If you are interested in having a mask that is fun to wear and fills others with joy when they see it, then you may want to buy one from Arm The Animals. These masks come in tiger face, dog face, cat face, and more. The company will also donate a mask to emergency workers, medical facilities, and California hospitals every time one is purchased.

- Amazon Handmade

Amazon Handmade is another great place to find cloth face masks. They work a lot like Etsy, in that they sell handmade items from people around the world. It is imperative that you make sure that you read the description of the face mask to make sure that you are getting one that is made of several cotton layers. If you are ordering during a time where there is a surge in need for face masks, a lot of these sellers may be at capacity. This means that it could take a month to get your shipment.

- eBay

Much like Etsy, eBay has lots of different sellers that offer reusable cloth face masks. eBay is a bit harder to sift through since the search for face mask tends to bring up outdoor activity masks and other face coverings as well, but you can find some that are suitable for your needs.

- American Blanket Company

The American Blanket Company is selling face masks made from fleece, which is a lot thicker than the standard face mask. They are also donating face masks to healthcare workers and first responders with every purchase that is made. You can purchase a five pack of masks for $39.

- Shami Oshun

Shami Oshun, historically, has been an independent fashion designer who makes 3d printings and color-changing fabrics. She is currently selling face masks that change colors in blue, pink, and purple for $38. The fabrics have been given a UV coating that gets activated in the sun and changes colors.

- Vera Bradley

While this may not be a brand you would expect to be on this list; Vera Bradley is manufacturing cloth face masks for $8 each. They are made with an opening for you to place disposable filters into to help keep out particles.

- Ask Local Groups

If you need face masks quickly and can't wait for items to be shipped out, you can always get in contact with social or religious groups that are close to you that you belong to, and see if they are making any that you could purchase.

When you are picking out your face mask, make sure you check what materials they use and how many layers. While layers are important, you don't want to choose one with so many layers that you can't breathe. It is important you are able to breathe through your mask. If you can't breathe through the mask, you will be taken in the air from around the mask. This means that you will be breathing in air that has not been filtered, and your nose hairs will hold onto tiny particles before they are sent deeper into your nose. That said, some materials may be too porous which allows for more particles to make it through the mask. Also, people have tried to use vacuum bags. These are tough to breathe through for humans, and some of them contain fiberglass, so under no circumstances should a vacuum filter be used.

A group of doctors and scientists at Wake Forest University recommends that a person holds their fabric options to a bright light and picking out ones where light cannot be seen through it. It is also been tested that using a double layer of cotton with at least a 180 thread count is good enough for a cloth face mask. Also, face masks that are made from a layer of regular cotton and then an inner layer of flannel works well.

Cambridge University compared the breathability and filtration of various types of homemade masks, and they discovered that masks created from cotton T-shirts or pillowcases struck the best balance.

As far as the shape of the mask, whether it is more of a cone shape or has an accordion fold, it doesn't really make a difference. Any type of facial covering is better than nothing at all. Plus, these are not medical masks so the pattern is not as important. The main thing is to make sure that they will fit over your nose and mouth and comes down over the chin and that they create as tight of a seal as possible. And I said this before, but it is imperative that you wash your cloth face mask before you wear.

Chapter 7: Other Ways to Protect Yourself

Microscopic organisms called pathogens cause infections. These can be parasites, fungi, viruses, or bacteria that get inside our bodies. Once inside, they will multiply, and interfere with our bodies normal functions. Diseases that are infectious are the main cause of death and illnesses in the world. For many people, especially those who have an underlying illness such as cancer or heart disease, people who have serious injuries, or ones who are taking medicines for a weak immune system, it is harder to stay away from getting an infection. Living in a country such as the United States, it is a very remote threat that we from parasites, bacteria, or deadly viruses. These microbes are always among us. Viruses and bacteria could be extremely contagious and make you sick. Nobody likes being sick, and there are things that could help you while battling germs.

You Have to Know How Infections Get Transmitted

It wasn't too long ago that nobody understood that diseases were caused by microscopic organisms that can be transmitted from person to person. Even though we now know the microscopic microbes can cause disease, the way they do isn't as obvious. We do understand that most of these microbes enter our bodies through body openings like our genitals, anuses, ears, mouths, and noses. They could be transmitted through the skin by an animal or insect bites. The easiest way to prevent getting infections is by stopping the pathogens from getting into the body.

Good Hygiene

This is your best line of defense when preventing infections. The first thing you have to do is to keep germs away from you by creating good hygiene habits. You have to prevent the infection before it starts and keep from spreading it to other people by following these easy steps.

- Wash Your Hands

This can't be said enough. Proper hygiene is the best way to prevent spreading infections. You might wash your hands after you use the bathroom, before you prepare food or eat, and after you have been feeding or petting animals, or gardening. You need to wash your hands after you sneeze, cough, or blow your nose or after you have cared or visited with someone who is sick. Wet your hands, lather well with soap, and rub this soap all over the backs and palms of your wrists and hands. Make sure you get in between your fingers, the backs and palms of your hands, and under your fingernails. Rinse well with running water. Dry your hands thoroughly.

- Cough Etiquette

You have to cover your nose and mouth when you sneeze or cough with either your elbow or tissue. If you do cover with a hand, make sure you wash your hands immediately with water and soap for at least 20 seconds. If you aren't near a water source, you can sanitize your hands using hand sanitizer.

- Injection Safety

This is a way to make sure that only one syringe and needle get used at one time. Injection safety has been associated with all the outbreaks of Hep B, and C. Never hesitate to ask your health care provider if they know about injection safety and if your syringe and needle should only be used one time.

- Sanitizing What's Around You

You need to follow any manufacturer's instructions when using any cleaning product. Each product will have a time frame that tells you how long a surface needs to stay wet for it to be properly cleaned. Some products like Clorox wipes tell you to leave it alone for four minutes or more. Make sure you protect your hands from these products, too.

- Other Precautions
    - If you get a cut, make sure to wash it thoroughly and put an appropriate bandage on it. Any human or animal bites need to be seen by a doctor. If the cut is serious or won't stop bleeding, see a doctor immediately.
    - Never squeeze a pimple. Don't pick at blemishes or wounds that are healing.
    - Don't pick up handkerchiefs, tissues, napkins, or other items that have been used by other people.
    - Never share eating utensils, glasses, or dishes.
- Antibiotic ABCs

Everyone needs to ask their doctors these questions when they want to prescribe an antibiotic:

- How do you know the type of infection I have because antibiotics don't work on viral infections?
- What side effects do I need to report to you?
- What drug interactions or side effects should I expect?
- Will this antibiotic help me get better?
- Do I actually need this antibiotic?

With some precautions and effort, you can make your life germ free and reduce your chances of getting an illness.

Practice Food Safety

Even though most cases of foodborne illnesses aren't dangerous, and some could lead to serious complications, including meningitis and kidney failure. There are ways to prevent these infections by storing and preparing your foods safely. The following will help you kill microbes that might be in your foods and keep you from introducing microbes to your food:

- Only defrost foods in the microwave or in the refrigerator.

- Thoroughly cook your food. Use a meat thermometer to make sure that ground meats are cooked to at least 160, steaks or roasts are at 145, and poultry is cooked to 180. Fish can be cooked until it turns opaque.

- Keep cooked foods and raw foods separated. Never use the same cutting boards or utensils for raw and cooked meats. Always wash the utensils or cutting boards between uses.

- Wash your hands, wash your hands, wash your hands.

- Seriously wash your hands anytime you handle meat that is raw.

- Rinse all vegetables and fruits before you serve them. Rinse fish, poultry, and meat under running water before cooking.

Vaccinations Are Essential

It doesn't matter if you are just young at heart or young; getting your vaccines is essential to staying healthy. Most infections could easily be prevented by getting your immunizations. Some vaccines can cause some side effects like a low grade fever or a sore arm but generally, they are very effective and safe.

Talk to your doctor about the status of your immunizations. Basically:

- Children need to receive their vaccines when they are due.

- If you an adult, you need to be sure your vaccines are up to date.

- When you are traveling to a different country, check with your doctor about any immunizations you might need to get before you go.

- Be sure that you are keeping your pet's vaccines up to date, as well. This won't just protect your pet, but it protects your family, too.

Travel Precautions

If you have planned on taking a trip, talk with your doctor about any immunizations that you might need. Talk about your travel plans with your doctor at least three months before you are scheduled to leave.

- Make sure to get the shots you need before you leave the US. Don't get any unnecessary shots, tattoos, or immunizations while overseas. Syringes and needles get reused in other parts of the world.

- If you are going to a place where there are a lot of insect borne diseases, take a good insect repellent that contains DEET. In most tropical regions, mosquitoes carry Japanese encephalitis, yellow fever, dengue, malaria, and other serious diseases.

- Only drink bottled drinks like bottled water or soft drinks. Make sure the caps are still sealed when you open them for the first time. Just be aware that some fruit juices are made with local water so they won't be pasteurized or uncontaminated.

- Never add ice to your drinks when traveling. Freezing won't kill waterborne microbes.

- Never consume any dairy products as the milk probably won't be pasteurized.

- Never eat uncooked veggies, including lettuce. Never eat fruit that you didn't peel yourself.

- All tap water needs to be boiled before you drink it or just drink bottled water. Make sure you use boiled or bottled water when you brush your teeth.

Sexually Transmitted Infections

The best way to make sure you don't transmit any sexual diseases is to just refrain from having any sexual contact or sexual intercourse. This isn't an option for most, so you need to follow these safe sex guidelines:

- Your partner and yourself need to be tested for HIV and other diseases that can be transmitted sexually.

- Only have sex with a partner that is only having sex with you.

If you do find a new partner, be sure they get tested and take these precautions:

- When engaging in anal sex, use a polyurethane or latex condom.

- When engaging in oral sex, use a polyurethane or latex condom for men or a female condom.

- When engaging in vaginal sex, use a polyurethane or latex condom or female condom.

Bug Borne Pathogens

Ticks and mosquitoes can carry various bacteria and viruses. Both have been cause some serious epidemics in the past decade.

Yes, it is true that most mosquitoes in the northern climates won't transmit diseases, but some can. In just ten years, the West Nile virus spread all across the US and into Canada. There are several more types of encephalitis that get carried by mosquitoes throughout North America. The tropical disease can be a threat if the mosquitoes that carry them hitch rides in boats or move out of Central America. The Zika virus was only found in the tropics but is now causing problems in Florida. Officials are worried that this illness might be creating a foothold in Florida since it has many marshlands and swamps. You have to make sure you keep yourself from getting mosquito bites as much as possible.

Ticks are pretty much everywhere and can give you various diseases like Lyme disease and encephalitis. They live in brushy and grassy areas and love wet seasons. They love to hide in wet leaves. They will usually infest animals like deer and field mice. They can be brought to your home on your pets.

To help prevent infections from bugs you need to:

- Look around your neighborhood and pick up any trash, throw away bottles, cans, and other containers that contain water that could let mosquitoes breed.

- Limit your outdoor activities during peak hours for mosquitoes, which are early evening and early morning.

- Keep any standing water drained near your house to keep the mosquito population down.

- Use an insect repellent that has been approved by the EPA, especially ones that contain eucalyptus essential oil, lemon essential oil, picaridin, or DEET. If mosquitoes keep biting you, keep applying the repellent.

- If a tick is attached to you or a pet, grasp it with tweezers close to its mouth and pull. Clean the area thoroughly with soap and water and wipe it down with some antiseptic. Watch the area for a few weeks for any signs of swelling or a rash.

- If you are planning on spending time in a place where ticks are common, wear clothing that is light colored so you can spot the tick and get rid of it before it attaches itself to you. If you are hiking, stay in the middle of the trail so you won't get any ticks from brush or bushes. Once you return, check your body and clothing for ticks. Always thoroughly check your pet before you bring it back inside.

Animal Control

You need to control how many rats or mice that live near your home. This can help you stay away from pathogens that are spread by rodents and can help control the population of ticks. Rodents can carry several pathogens that include hantavirus, plague, leptospirosis, and lymphocytic choriomeningitis virus. There are other wild animals that could transmit rabies or other diseases. You can do the following to help you stay away from getting sick from a disease brought to you by a wild animal:

- Stay away from wild animals. Most wild animals like coyotes, foxes, bats, skunks, and raccoons can spread rabies to humans through a bite. Try to keep your pets away from them also. Cats, dogs, and any other warm-blooded animal can get rabies from a wild animal. Rabies can be passed to humans, too.

- If you have a severe rodent problem, you should talk to a pest control professional.

- If you are outdoors, don't handle or disturb rodent dens or burrows.

- Never stir up dust in any area that is infested with rodents. Use a sponge or wet mop that has been wet down with disinfectant.

- Clear all junk or brush away from your home's foundation.

- Seal all cracks and holes in your house to close off their access inside your home.

- All garbage and food needs to stay covered and in a container that is rodent proof.

Coronavirus or COVID-19

The first thing you should know is the way this spreads. It is spread from person to person between people who are in close contact with others. This means closer than six feet.

It can be transmitted through droplets that get produced when a person who is infected talks, sneezes, or coughs. The droplets could land in the nose or mouth of anyone who is close by. It can be inhaled into their lungs, too.

Some studies show that COVID-19 might spread by a person who isn't even showing any signs or symptoms.

The best way to keep from getting this disease is to not be exposed to the virus.

There aren't any vaccines that can prevent COVID-19 right now.

Everybody Needs to

You need to make sure you clean your hands as often as you possibly can. Wash them with water and soap for 20 seconds, especially if you have been out in public or after you have sneezed, coughed, or blew your nose. Make sure you get in between your fingers and under your fingernails.

If you don't have water and soap handy, you can use hand sanitizer that is at least 60 percent alcohol. Make sure you cover every surface of your hands and rub until they are dry.

Try your best not to touch your mouth, nose, or eyes until you have washed your hands.

Keep Your Distance

If you know someone who is sick, stay away from them if you can. If not, try to wear a mask and wash your hands as soon as you leave them. If you are able to, try to keep at least six feet between them and you.

Try your best to stay at home as much as you possibly can.

If you have to go out for groceries or to pick up a prescription, try your best to keep as much distance as you can between yourself and others. You have to keep in mind that some people who aren't showing any symptoms might still be able to spread the virus if they have been near someone who has it.

Keeping at least six feet between you and others is very important if you are at a high risk of getting sick.

Try to wear a cloth face mask when you are around other people. You might spread COVID-19 to other people even when you don't feel sick.

Face Masks

You should wear a cloth face mask when you need to go out to get groceries or a prescription. Remember to not put a face mask on children who are younger than two years, anybody who has trouble breathing, is incapacitated or unconscious, or can remove the mask without having help.

This face mask is being used to protect others if you think you have been infected or have been around others who are infected. Don't buy or use face masks that are intended for health care workers.

Always keep six feet between yourself and others. The face mask isn't meant to replace social distancing.

Sneezes and Coughs

Make sure you always cover your sneezes and coughs. Wherever you may be and if you don't have on a face mask, always cover your nose and mouth with a tissue or sneeze and cough into the inside of your elbow or down the front of your shirt.

Immediately throw the tissue into the trash.

Wash your hands with water and soap for 20 seconds as quickly as you can after you cough. If you aren't near water and soap, use a hand sanitizer.

Disinfecting and Cleaning

Make sure you disinfect and clean all surfaces that are touched frequently each day. This includes sinks, faucets, toilets, keyboards, phones, desks, handles, countertops, light switches, doorknobs, and tables.

If you can see dirt on any surface, clean it immediately. Use water and soap or a spray cleaner before you disinfect the surface.

To disinfect, the EPA says that any registered household disinfectant is going to work. Use it appropriately for the surface you are cleaning.

- Disinfectant Options

There are other options out there that you can use to clean your house. Just know that if you have pets, some of these might be toxic to your pet. Please, please check with your vet before you clean with something that might harm your pet.

To make a bleach solution, you are going to mix five tablespoons of bleach to one gallon of water. You could also use four teaspoons in a quart of water.

Follow the manufacturer's instructions when using bleach and make sure your space is properly ventilated. Make sure the product isn't past the expiration date. Never mix ammonia and bleach. Basically, don't mix bleach with any other household cleaner. Bleach that isn't expired is very effective against the coronavirus if it is diluted correctly.

If you want to use alcohol in any solution, make sure the alcohol is at least 70 percent alcohol.

All household disinfectants that have been registered with the EPA are good at killing viruses. Just follow the manufacturer's instructions when you are disinfecting and cleaning things.

Conclusion

Thank you for making it through to the end of the book, and I hope it was informative and able to provide you with all of the tools you need to achieve your goals whatever they may be.

The next step is to try making some face masks for yourself. You never know when the time may come that you need to use a face mask to protect yourself or others. Making the face masks could also be something you do for charity when there is a need for it. Above all else, always practice good hygiene to help prevent the spread of disease.

Finally, if you found this book useful in any way, a review on Amazon is always appreciated!

www.ingramcontent.com/pod-product-compliance
Lightning Source LLC
Chambersburg PA
CBHW081811240526
45465CB00032BA/2797